Blood Pressure Log

Month & Year ______________________________

Week Starting ______________________________

Weight ______________________________

Date	Time	Systolic	Diastolic	Heart Rate	Notes

Blood Pressure Log

Month & Year ______________________

Week Starting ______________________

Weight ______________________

Date	Time	Systolic	Diastolic	Heart Rate	Notes

Blood Pressure Log

Month & Year ______________________

Week Starting ______________________

Weight ______________________

Date	Time	Systolic	Diastolic	Heart Rate	Notes

Blood Pressure Log

Month & Year ____________________

Week Starting ____________________

Weight ____________________

Date	Time	Systolic	Diastolic	Heart Rate	Notes

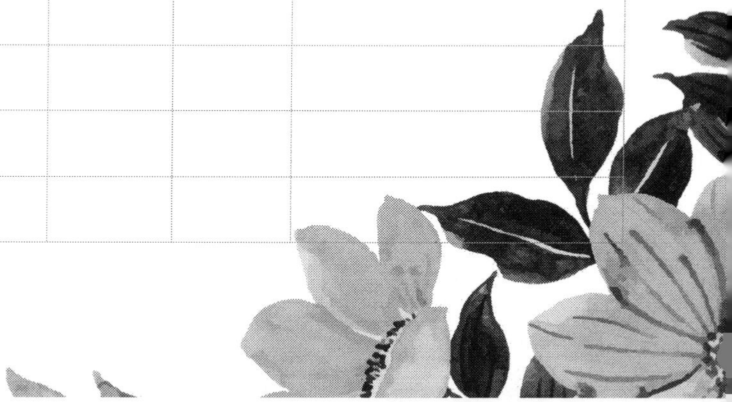

Blood Pressure Log

Month & Year ______________________________

Week Starting ______________________________

Weight ______________________________

Date	Time	Systolic	Diastolic	Heart Rate	Notes

Blood Pressure Log

Month & Year ______________________________

Week Starting ______________________________

Weight ______________________________

Date	Time	Systolic	Diastolic	Heart Rate	Notes

Blood Pressure Log

Month & Year ______________________

Week Starting ______________________

Weight ______________________

Date	Time	Systolic	Diastolic	Heart Rate	Notes

Blood Pressure Log

Month & Year ______________________________

Week Starting ______________________________

Weight ______________________________

Date	Time	Systolic	Diastolic	Heart Rate	Notes

Blood Pressure Log

Month & Year ______________________________

Week Starting ______________________________

Weight ______________________________

Date	Time	Systolic	Diastolic	Heart Rate	Notes

Blood Pressure Log

Month & Year ______________________________

Week Starting ______________________________

Weight ______________________________

Date	Time	Systolic	Diastolic	Heart Rate	Notes

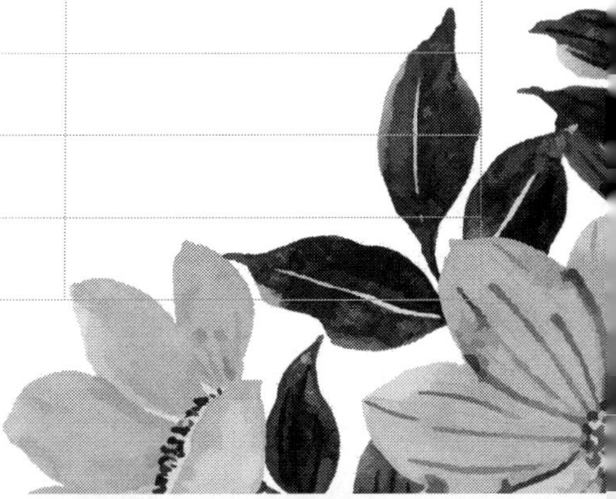

Blood Pressure Log

Month & Year ______________________

Week Starting ______________________

Weight ______________________

Date	Time	Systolic	Diastolic	Heart Rate	Notes

Blood Pressure Log

Month & Year ______________________

Week Starting ______________________

Weight ______________________

Date	Time	Systolic	Diastolic	Heart Rate	Notes

Blood Pressure Log

Month & Year ______________________________

Week Starting ______________________________

Weight ______________________________

Date	Time	Systolic	Diastolic	Heart Rate	Notes

Blood Pressure Log

Month & Year ____________________

Week Starting ____________________

Weight ____________________

Date	Time	Systolic	Diastolic	Heart Rate	Notes

Blood Pressure Log

Month & Year ____________________

Week Starting ____________________

Weight ____________________

Date	Time	Systolic	Diastolic	Heart Rate	Notes

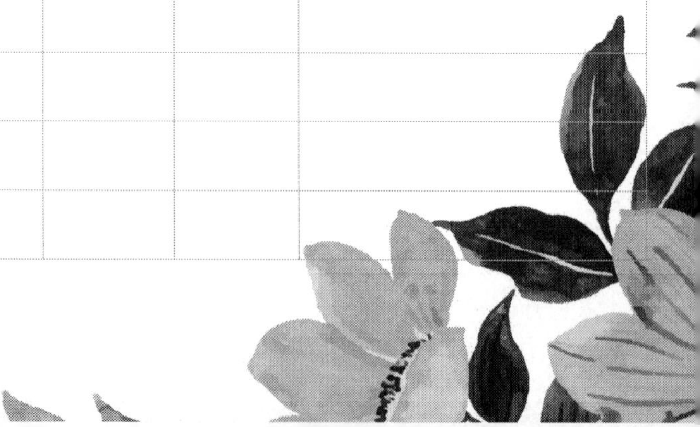

Blood Pressure Log

Month & Year ______________________

Week Starting ______________________

Weight ______________________

Date	Time	Systolic	Diastolic	Heart Rate	Notes

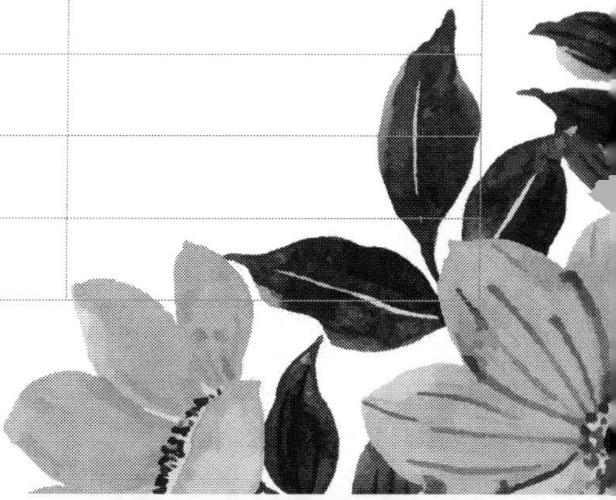

Blood Pressure Log

Month & Year ______________________

Week Starting ______________________

Weight ______________________

Date	Time	Systolic	Diastolic	Heart Rate	Notes

Blood Pressure Log

Month & Year ____________________

Week Starting ____________________

Weight ____________________

Date	Time	Systolic	Diastolic	Heart Rate	Notes

Blood Pressure Log

Month & Year ______________________________

Week Starting ______________________________

Weight ______________________________

Date	Time	Systolic	Diastolic	Heart Rate	Notes

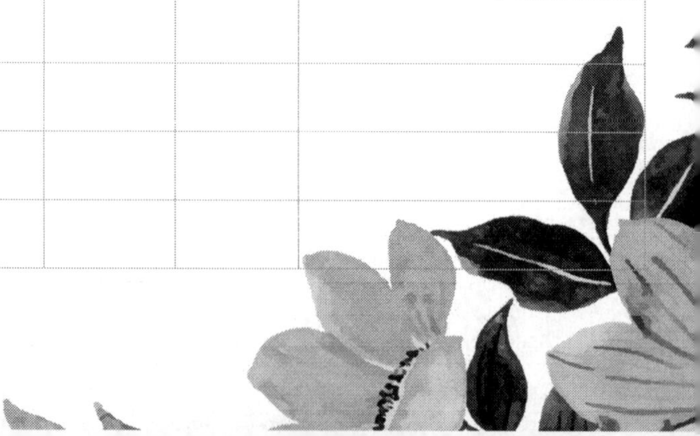

Blood Pressure Log

Month & Year ______________________________

Week Starting ______________________________

Weight ______________________________

Date	Time	Systolic	Diastolic	Heart Rate	Notes

Blood Pressure Log

Month & Year ______________________________

Week Starting ______________________________

Weight ______________________________

Date	Time	Systolic	Diastolic	Heart Rate	Notes

Blood Pressure Log

Month & Year ______________________

Week Starting ______________________

Weight ______________________

Date	Time	Systolic	Diastolic	Heart Rate	Notes

Blood Pressure Log

Month & Year ______________________________

Week Starting ______________________________

Weight ______________________________

Date	Time	Systolic	Diastolic	Heart Rate	Notes

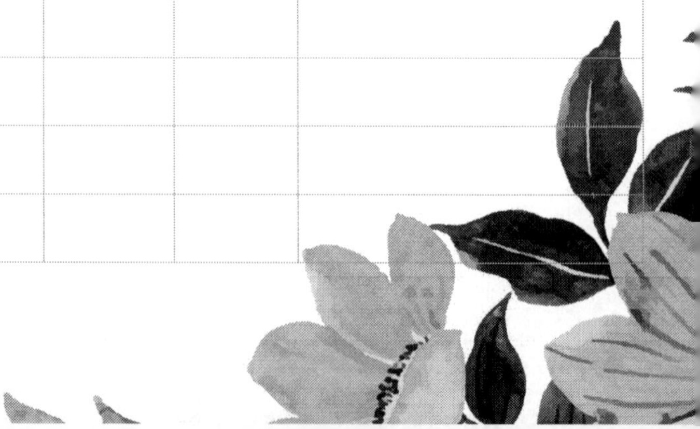

Blood Pressure Log

Month & Year ______________________

Week Starting ______________________

Weight ______________________

Date	Time	Systolic	Diastolic	Heart Rate	Notes

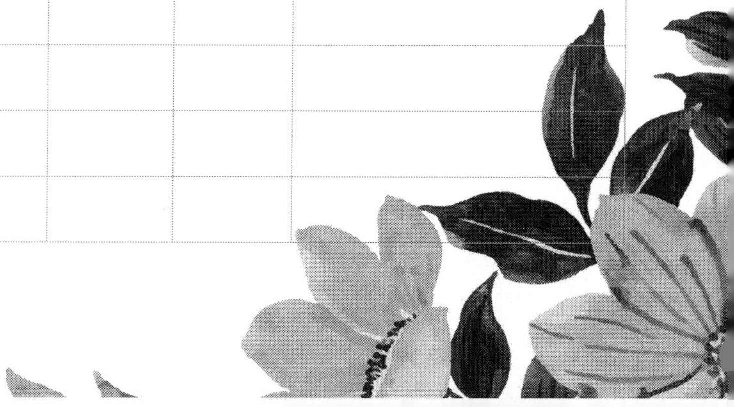

Blood Pressure Log

Month & Year ______________________________

Week Starting ______________________________

Weight ______________________________

Date	Time	Systolic	Diastolic	Heart Rate	Notes

Blood Pressure Log

Month & Year ______________________________

Week Starting ______________________________

Weight ______________________________

Date	Time	Systolic	Diastolic	Heart Rate	Notes

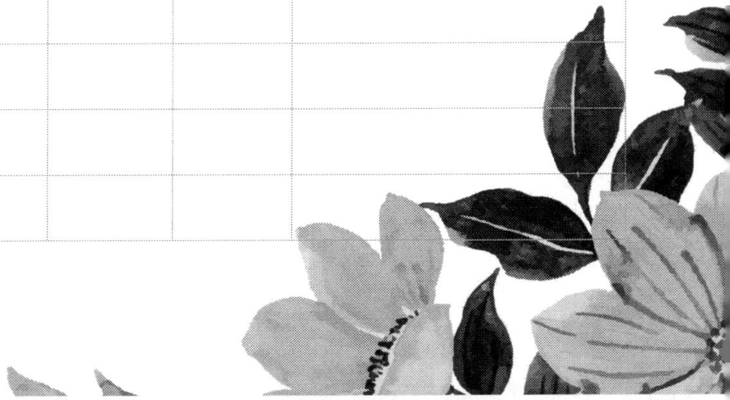

Blood Pressure Log

Month & Year ______________________

Week Starting ______________________

Weight ______________________

Date	Time	Systolic	Diastolic	Heart Rate	Notes

Blood Pressure Log

Month & Year ____________________

Week Starting ____________________

Weight ____________________

Date	Time	Systolic	Diastolic	Heart Rate	Notes

Blood Pressure Log

Month & Year ______________________________

Week Starting ______________________________

Weight ______________________________

Date	Time	Systolic	Diastolic	Heart Rate	Notes

Blood Pressure Log

Month & Year ______________________________

Week Starting ______________________________

Weight ______________________________

Date	Time	Systolic	Diastolic	Heart Rate	Notes

Blood Pressure Log

Month & Year ______________________________

Week Starting ______________________________

Weight ______________________________

Date	Time	Systolic	Diastolic	Heart Rate	Notes

Blood Pressure Log

Month & Year ____________________

Week Starting ____________________

Weight ____________________

Date	Time	Systolic	Diastolic	Heart Rate	Notes

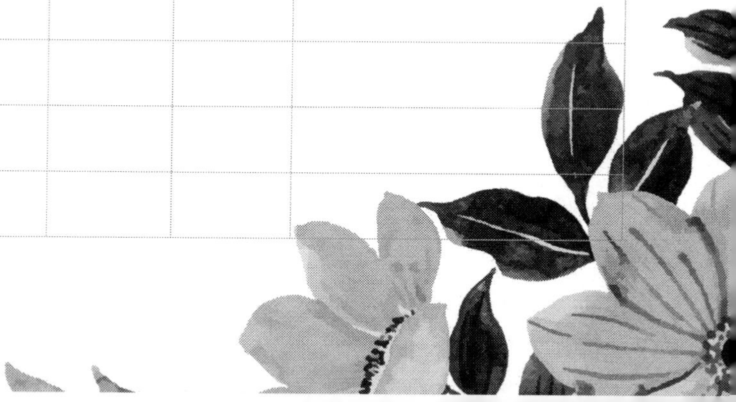

Blood Pressure Log

Month & Year ______________________

Week Starting ______________________

Weight ______________________

Date	Time	Systolic	Diastolic	Heart Rate	Notes

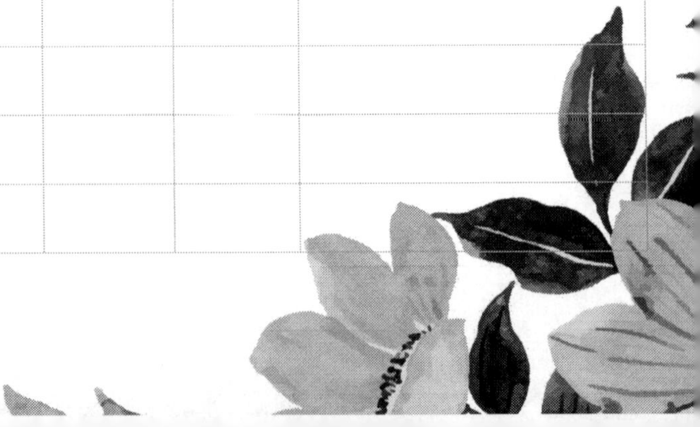

Blood Pressure Log

Month & Year ____________________

Week Starting ____________________

Weight ____________________

Date	Time	Systolic	Diastolic	Heart Rate	Notes

Blood Pressure Log

Month & Year ______________________________

Week Starting ______________________________

Weight ______________________________

Date	Time	Systolic	Diastolic	Heart Rate	Notes

Blood Pressure Log

Month & Year ______________________

Week Starting ______________________

Weight ______________________

Date	Time	Systolic	Diastolic	Heart Rate	Notes

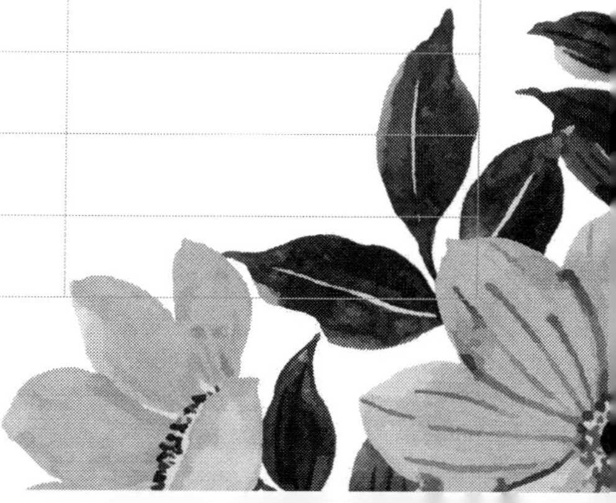

Blood Pressure Log

Month & Year ____________________

Week Starting ____________________

Weight ____________________

Date	Time	Systolic	Diastolic	Heart Rate	Notes

Blood Pressure Log

Month & Year ______________________

Week Starting ______________________

Weight ______________________

Date	Time	Systolic	Diastolic	Heart Rate	Notes

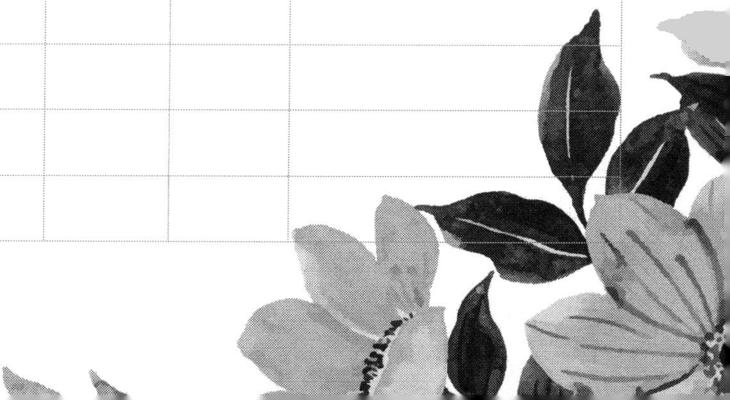

Blood Pressure Log

Month & Year ______________________________

Week Starting ______________________________

Weight ______________________________

Date	Time	Systolic	Diastolic	Heart Rate	Notes

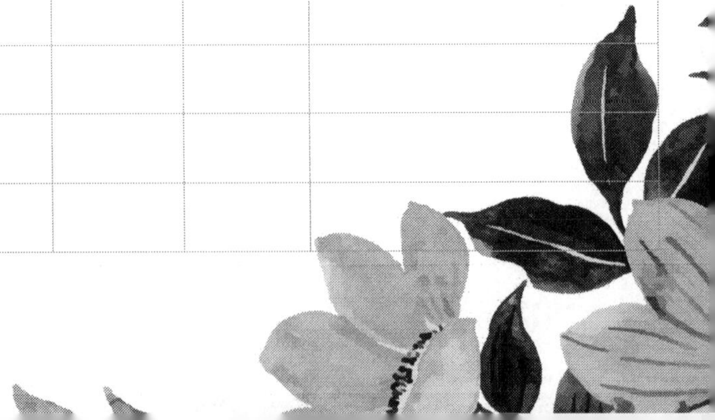

Blood Pressure Log

Month & Year ______________________

Week Starting ______________________

Weight ______________________

Date	Time	Systolic	Diastolic	Heart Rate	Notes

Blood Pressure Log

Month & Year ______________________________

Week Starting ______________________________

Weight ______________________________

Date	Time	Systolic	Diastolic	Heart Rate	Notes

Blood Pressure Log

Month & Year ______________________

Week Starting ______________________

Weight ______________________

Date	Time	Systolic	Diastolic	Heart Rate	Notes

Blood Pressure Log

Month & Year ______________________

Week Starting ______________________

Weight ______________________

Date	Time	Systolic	Diastolic	Heart Rate	Notes

Blood Pressure Log

Month & Year ______________________________

Week Starting ______________________________

Weight ______________________________

Date	Time	Systolic	Diastolic	Heart Rate	Notes

Blood Pressure Log

Month & Year ______________________________

Week Starting ______________________________

Weight ______________________________

Date	Time	Systolic	Diastolic	Heart Rate	Notes

Blood Pressure Log

Month & Year ______________________________

Week Starting ______________________________

Weight ______________________________

Date	Time	Systolic	Diastolic	Heart Rate	Notes

Blood Pressure Log

Month & Year ______________________________

Week Starting ______________________________

Weight ______________________________

Date	Time	Systolic	Diastolic	Heart Rate	Notes

Blood Pressure Log

Month & Year ____________________

Week Starting ____________________

Weight ____________________

Date	Time	Systolic	Diastolic	Heart Rate	Notes

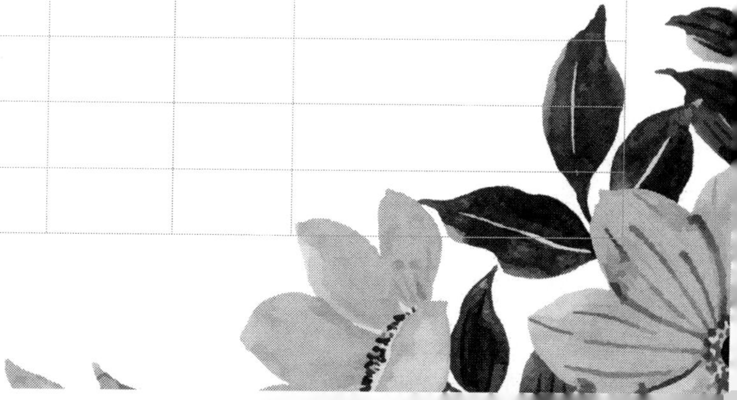

Blood Pressure Log

Month & Year ______________________

Week Starting ______________________

Weight ______________________

Date	Time	Systolic	Diastolic	Heart Rate	Notes

Blood Pressure Log

Month & Year ______________________________

Week Starting ______________________________

Weight ______________________________

Date	Time	Systolic	Diastolic	Heart Rate	Notes

Blood Pressure Log

Month & Year ______________________________

Week Starting ______________________________

Weight ______________________________

Date	Time	Systolic	Diastolic	Heart Rate	Notes

Blood Pressure Log

Month & Year ______________________________

Week Starting ______________________________

Weight ______________________________

Date	Time	Systolic	Diastolic	Heart Rate	Notes

Blood Pressure Log

Month & Year ______________________________

Week Starting ______________________________

Weight ______________________________

Date	Time	Systolic	Diastolic	Heart Rate	Notes

Blood Pressure Log

Month & Year ______________________________

Week Starting ______________________________

Weight ______________________________

Date	Time	Systolic	Diastolic	Heart Rate	Notes

Blood Pressure Log

Month & Year ____________________

Week Starting ____________________

Weight ____________________

Date	Time	Systolic	Diastolic	Heart Rate	Notes

Blood Pressure Log

Month & Year ______________________________

Week Starting ______________________________

Weight ______________________________

Date	Time	Systolic	Diastolic	Heart Rate	Notes

Blood Pressure Log

Month & Year ______________________

Week Starting ______________________

Weight ______________________

Date	Time	Systolic	Diastolic	Heart Rate	Notes

Blood Pressure Log

Month & Year ______________________________

Week Starting ______________________________

Weight ______________________________

Date	Time	Systolic	Diastolic	Heart Rate	Notes

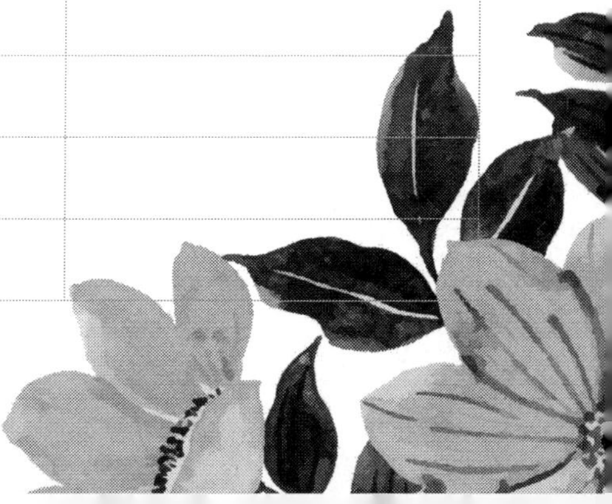

Blood Pressure Log

Month & Year ______________________________

Week Starting ______________________________

Weight ______________________________

Date	Time	Systolic	Diastolic	Heart Rate	Notes

Blood Pressure Log

Month & Year ______________________________

Week Starting ______________________________

Weight ______________________________

Date	Time	Systolic	Diastolic	Heart Rate	Notes

Blood Pressure Log

Month & Year ____________________

Week Starting ____________________

Weight ____________________

Date	Time	Systolic	Diastolic	Heart Rate	Notes

Blood Pressure Log

Month & Year ______________________

Week Starting ______________________

Weight ______________________

Date	Time	Systolic	Diastolic	Heart Rate	Notes

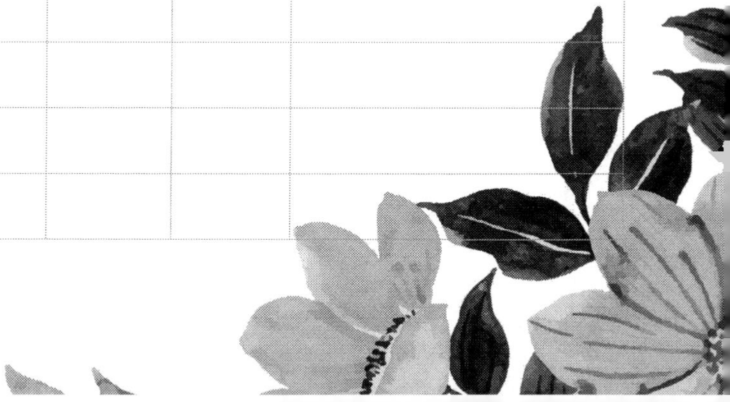

Blood Pressure Log

Month & Year ______________________

Week Starting ______________________

Weight ______________________

Date	Time	Systolic	Diastolic	Heart Rate	Notes

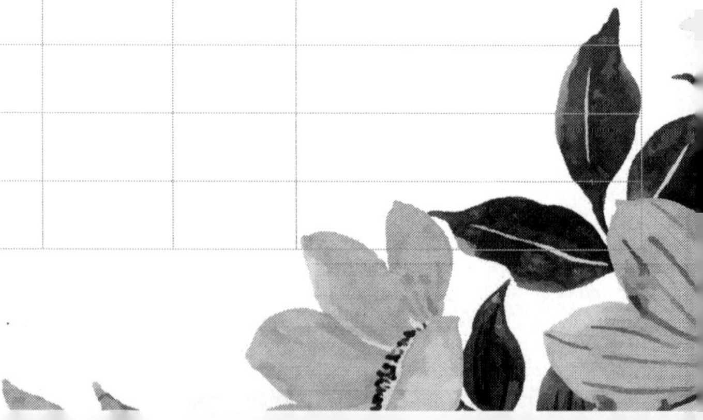

Blood Pressure Log

Month & Year ______________________________

Week Starting ______________________________

Weight ______________________________

Date	Time	Systolic	Diastolic	Heart Rate	Notes

Blood Pressure Log

Month & Year ______________________

Week Starting ______________________

Weight ______________________

Date	Time	Systolic	Diastolic	Heart Rate	Notes

Blood Pressure Log

Month & Year ______________________________

Week Starting ______________________________

Weight ______________________________

Date	Time	Systolic	Diastolic	Heart Rate	Notes

Blood Pressure Log

Month & Year ______________________

Week Starting ______________________

Weight ______________________

Date	Time	Systolic	Diastolic	Heart Rate	Notes

Blood Pressure Log

Month & Year ____________________

Week Starting ____________________

Weight ____________________

Date	Time	Systolic	Diastolic	Heart Rate	Notes

Blood Pressure Log

Month & Year ______________________________

Week Starting ______________________________

Weight ______________________________

Date	Time	Systolic	Diastolic	Heart Rate	Notes

Blood Pressure Log

Month & Year ______________________

Week Starting ______________________

Weight ______________________

Date	Time	Systolic	Diastolic	Heart Rate	Notes

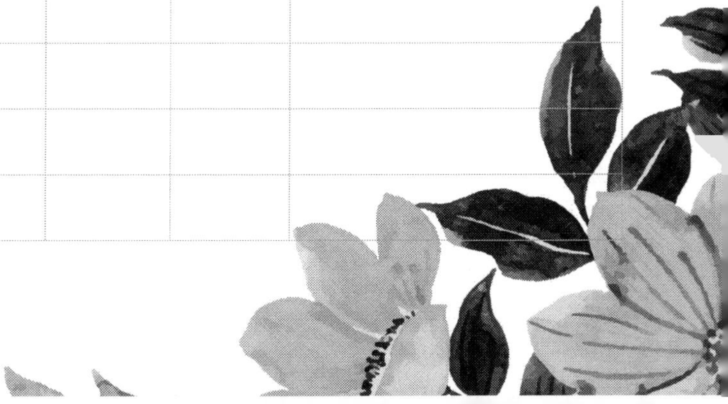

Blood Pressure Log

Month & Year ______________________

Week Starting ______________________

Weight ______________________

Date	Time	Systolic	Diastolic	Heart Rate	Notes

Blood Pressure Log

Month & Year ______________________________

Week Starting ______________________________

Weight ______________________________

Date	Time	Systolic	Diastolic	Heart Rate	Notes

Blood Pressure Log

Month & Year ______________________________

Week Starting ______________________________

Weight ______________________________

Date	Time	Systolic	Diastolic	Heart Rate	Notes

Blood Pressure Log

Month & Year ______________________

Week Starting ______________________

Weight ______________________

Date	Time	Systolic	Diastolic	Heart Rate	Notes

Blood Pressure Log

Month & Year ______________________

Week Starting ______________________

Weight ______________________

Date	Time	Systolic	Diastolic	Heart Rate	Notes

Blood Pressure Log

Month & Year ______________________________

Week Starting ______________________________

Weight ______________________________

Date	Time	Systolic	Diastolic	Heart Rate	Notes

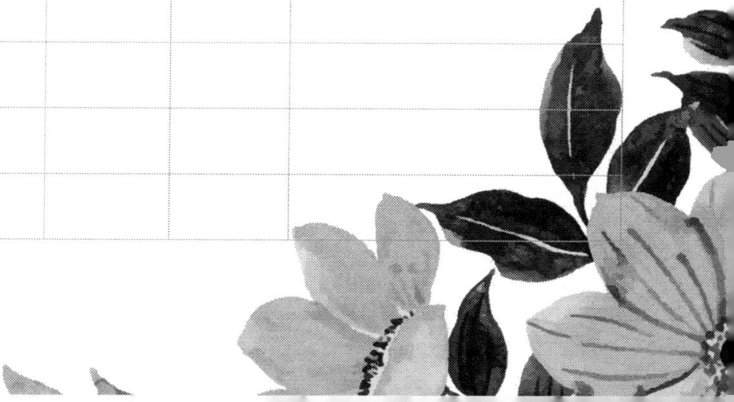

Blood Pressure Log

Month & Year ____________________

Week Starting ____________________

Weight ____________________

Date	Time	Systolic	Diastolic	Heart Rate	Notes

Blood Pressure Log

Month & Year ______________________

Week Starting ______________________

Weight ______________________

Date	Time	Systolic	Diastolic	Heart Rate	Notes

Blood Pressure Log

Month & Year ______________________________

Week Starting ______________________________

Weight ______________________________

Date	Time	Systolic	Diastolic	Heart Rate	Notes

Blood Pressure Log

Month & Year ______________________

Week Starting ______________________

Weight ______________________

Date	Time	Systolic	Diastolic	Heart Rate	Notes

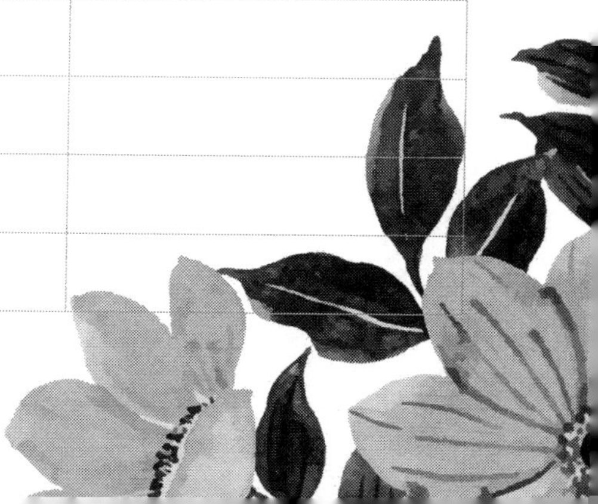

Made in United States
Troutdale, OR
11/03/2026

56844453R00046